MY "I AM" BOOK
AFIRMATIONS JOURNAL

Priscilla Mills

INTRODUCTION

Since very young age, we spend days learning and observing general life passing through. We grab information and we assume on how events may happen around us, creating believes that can be far away from our own reality.

Allow yourself to receive the great abundance that surrender you!

In this book we are offering practical daily exercises as a guidance to re-programme your mind with positive affirmations. We offer 30 days of powerful affirmations to practice every day, giving you the chance to interact adding your preferences and following your progress on your own peace.

Repeating affirmations helps to reprogram the unconscious mind for success. The brain takes around 28 days to start reprogramming our believes, through constancy, repetition, visualization and emotional feelings.

Remember, what you think, say, or feel becomes your reality!

Affirmations are short, powerful, yet simple statements designed to help you manifest your desires.

Start this amazing journey day by day and open your mind to see the changes coming!

Priscilla Mills

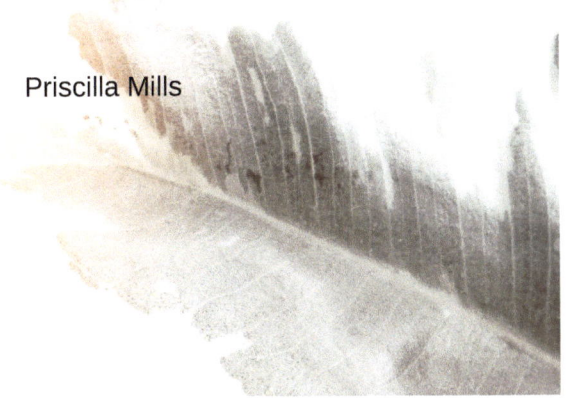

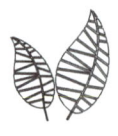 # A Step-By-Step Guide

- It is important that before starting your journal you find a peaceful and comfortable place to read out loud the affirmations.

- Remember to repeat each paragraph at least 5 times, twice a day. Once when you first arise in the morning, and once right before bed-time. Feel free to do more if desire.

- While doing this make sure you are attaching positive emotions to each word. Think about how achieving your goal will make you feel and make sure to continually flood your subconscious with thoughts and images of the new reality you wish to create.

- Remember to stay focused on your goals and to come up with solutions to challenges and obstacles that might get in the way.

- Keep present that the affirmations are for yourself, not others.

Make them powerful and unique!

DAY 1

**Find a peaceful place to read out loud the affirmations.
Repeat each paragraph 5 times, twice a day.**

I am healthy.
I am healthy.
I am healthy.

I am worthy of love and deserve to receive love in abundance.
I am worthy of love and deserve to receive love in abundance.
I am worthy of love and deserve to receive love in abundance.

I am beautiful and my body regenerates and revitalises every second
of my life.
I am beautiful and my body regenerates and revitalises every second
of my life.
I am beautiful and my body regenerates and revitalises every second
of my life.

Write your own:

I am _____

I am _____

I am _____

I am _____

I am _____

I am _____

I am _____

DAY 2

Find a peaceful place to read out loud the affirmations.
Repeat each paragraph 5 times, twice a day.

I am wealthy and prosperous.
I am wealthy and prosperous.
I am wealthy and prosperous.

I am fearless, I am brave and capable to achieve anything I want.
I am fearless, I am brave and capable to achieve anything I want.
I am fearless, I am brave and capable to achieve anything I want.

I am in perfect health. Wellness is the natural state of my body.
I am in perfect health. Wellness is the natural state of my body.
I am in perfect health. Wellness is the natural state of my body.

Write your own:

I am _____

I am _____

I am _____

I am _____

I am _____

I am _____

I am _____

DAY 3

**Find a peaceful place to read out loud the affirmations.
Repeat each paragraph 5 times, twice a day.**

I am a magnet to attract great people into my life.
I am a magnet to attract great people into my life.
I am a magnet to attract great people into my life.

I am beautiful. I am strong. I am powerful.
I am beautiful. I am strong. I am powerful.
I am beautiful. I am strong. I am powerful.

I am grateful for my family, I am grateful for my life, I am grateful for
all my achievements.
I am grateful for my family, I am grateful for my life, I am grateful for
all my achievements.
I am grateful for my family, I am grateful for my life, I am grateful for
all my achievements.

Write your own:

I am _____

I am _____

I am _____

I am _____

I am _____

I am _____

I am _____

DAY 4

**Find a peaceful place to read out loud the affirmations.
Repeat each paragraph 5 times, twice a day.**

I am a magnet to attract great opportunities in my live.
I am a magnet to attract great opportunities in my live.
I am a magnet to attract great opportunities in my live.

I am in control of my life and my circumstances.
I am in control of my life and my circumstances.
I am in control of my life and my circumstances.

I am eating healthy food and choosing carefully my diet.
I am eating healthy food and choosing carefully my diet.
I am eating healthy food and choosing carefully my diet.

Write your own:

I am _____

I am _____

I am _____

I am _____

I am _____

I am _____

I am _____

Remember to Visualise

DAY 5

**Find a peaceful place to read out loud the affirmations.
Repeat each paragraph 5 times, twice a day.**

I am feeling more happy, healthier and peaceful every day.
I am feeling more happy, healthier and peaceful every day.
I am feeling more happy, healthier and peaceful every day.

I am respectful, kind and worthy of true love.
I am respectful, kind and worthy of true love.
I am respectful, kind and worthy of true love.

I am prosperous and abundant. The universe is always aligned in my favour.
I am prosperous and abundant. The universe is always aligned in my favour.
I am prosperous and abundant. The universe is always aligned in my favour.

Write your own:

I am _____

I am _____

I am _____

I am _____

I am _____

I am _____

I am _____

DAY 6

**Find a peaceful place to read out loud the affirmations.
Repeat each paragraph 5 times, twice a day.**

I am worthy of love, respect and true friendships.
I am worthy of love, respect and true friendships.
I am worthy of love, respect and true friendships.

I am strong, and I grow stronger every day.
I am strong, and I grow stronger every day.
I am strong, and I grow stronger every day.

I am young and my body regenerates and revitalises every day.
I am young and my body regenerates and revitalises every day.
I am young and my body regenerates and revitalises every day.

Write your own:

I am _____

I am _____

I am _____

I am _____

I am _____

I am _____

I am _____

Remember to Visualise

DAY 7

**Find a peaceful place to read out loud the affirmations.
Repeat each paragraph 5 times, twice a day.**

I am important and a valuable person.
I am important and a valuable person.
I am important and a valuable person.

I am manifesting new and exciting opportunities.
I am manifesting new and exciting opportunities.
I am manifesting new and exciting opportunities.

I am always receiving good news.
I am always receiving good news.
I am always receiving good news.

Write your own:

I am _____

I am _____

I am _____

I am _____

I am _____

I am _____

I am _____

DAY 8

Find a peaceful place to read out loud the affirmations.
Repeat each paragraph 5 times, twice a day.

I am safe. I am in control. I am powerful.
I am safe. I am in control. I am powerful.
I am safe. I am in control. I am powerful.

I am constantly attracting abundance and money.
I am constantly attracting abundance and money.
I am constantly attracting abundance and money.

I am resilient and can handle problems with expertise.
I am resilient and can handle problems with expertise.
I am resilient and can handle problems with expertise.

Write your own:

I am _____

I am _____

I am _____

I am _____

I am _____

I am _____

I am _____

DAY 9

Find a peaceful place to read out loud the affirmations.
Repeat each paragraph 5 times, twice a day.

II am amazing, and everybody loves me.
I am amazing, and everybody loves me.
I am amazing, and everybody loves me.

I am so happy of feeding myself with healthy food.
I am so happy of feeding myself with healthy food.
I am so happy of feeding myself with healthy food.

I am so happy and grateful that I am now earning £_____a year.
I am so happy and grateful that I am now earning £_____a year.
I am so happy and grateful that I am now earning £_____a year.

Write your own:

I am _____

I am _____

I am _____

I am _____

I am _____

I am _____

I am _____

Remember to Visualise

DAY 10

**Find a peaceful place to read out loud the affirmations.
Repeat each paragraph 5 times, twice a day.**

I am grateful for who I am and can be.
I am grateful for who I am and can be.
I am grateful for who I am and can be.

I am on the right path. I am moving in the right direction.
I am on the right path. I am moving in the right direction.
I am on the right path. I am moving in the right direction.

I am abundant, confident and inspired.
I am abundant, confident and inspired.
I am abundant, confident and inspired.

Write your own:

I am _____

I am _____

I am _____

I am _____

I am _____

I am _____

I am _____

REVIEW YOUR PROGRESS

Well done! This has been 10 days since you started to reprogram your mind with powerful positive affirmations.

Remember to be consistent. When changes are needed in your life, it should all start with your thoughts. When you repeat an affirmation to yourself, it should be out-loud or in your mind, your mind is re-trained to begin to see these affirmations as absolute truth.

Count your blessings and write down your achievements.

_____

_____

_____

_____

_____

DAY 11

**Find a peaceful place to read out loud the affirmations.
Repeat each paragraph 5 times, twice a day.**

I am powerful and capable of anything I set my mind to.
I am powerful and capable of anything I set my mind to.
I am powerful and capable of anything I set my mind to.

I am in a great health and my body cells regenerate every second of my life.
I am in a great health and my body cells regenerate every second of my life.
I am in a great health and my body cells regenerate every second of my life.

I am safe, I am protected and in control.
I am safe, I am protected and in control.
I am safe, I am protected and in control.

Write your own:

I am _____

I am _____

I am _____

I am _____

I am _____

I am _____

I am _____

Remember to Visualise

DAY 12

**Find a peaceful place to read out loud the affirmations.
Repeat each paragraph 5 times, twice a day.**

I am an amazing human being and I deserve happiness, love,
prosperity and health.
I am an amazing human being and I deserve happiness, love,
prosperity and health.
I am an amazing human being and I deserve happiness, love,
prosperity and health.

I am receiving wellness now in my life.
I am receiving wellness now in my life.
I am receiving wellness now in my life.

I am always positive about myself. I am exceptional and motivated.
I am always positive about myself. I am exceptional and motivated.
I am always positive about myself. I am exceptional and motivated.

Write your own:

I am _____

I am _____

I am _____

I am _____

I am _____

I am _____

I am _____

DAY 13

**Find a peaceful place to read out loud the affirmations.
Repeat each paragraph 5 times, twice a day.**

I am attracting great and positive people every day.
I am attracting great and positive people every day.
I am attracting great and positive people every day.

I am worthy of all good things.
I am worthy of all good things.
I am worthy of all good things.

I am good looking, attractive, kind and powerful.
I am good looking, attractive, kind and powerful.
I am good looking, attractive, kind and powerful.

Write your own:

I am _____

I am _____

I am _____

I am _____

I am _____

I am _____

I am _____

Remember to Visualise

DAY 14

**Find a peaceful place to read out loud the affirmations.
Repeat each paragraph 5 times, twice a day.**

I am successfully changing my mindset positively.
I am successful changing my mindset positively.
I am successful changing my mindset positively.

I am vibrating in harmony and prosperity.
I am vibrating in harmony and prosperity.
I am vibrating in harmony and prosperity.

I am radiant in love and health every second.
I am radiant in love and health every second.
I am radiant in love and health every second.

Write your own:

I am _____

I am _____

I am _____

I am _____

I am _____

I am _____

I am _____

DAY 15

Find a peaceful place to read out loud the affirmations.
Repeat each paragraph 5 times, twice a day.

II am respectful, respected and admired.
I am respectful, respected and admired.
I am respectful, respected and admired.

I am attracting money and wealthiest into my life.
I am attracting money and wealthiest into my life.
I am attracting money and wealthiest into my life.

I am a winner. I am capable of achieving anything I want.
I am a winner. I am capable of achieving anything I want.
I am a winner. I am capable of achieving anything I want.

Write your own:

I am _____

I am _____

I am _____

I am _____

I am _____

I am _____

I am _____

DAY 16

**Find a peaceful place to read out loud the affirmations.
Repeat each paragraph 5 times, twice a day.**

I am assertive, and open to listen to others.
I am assertive, and open to listen to others.
I am assertive, and open to listen to others.

I am in peace and in control of my feelings.
I am in peace and in control of my feelings.
I am in peace and in control of my feelings.

I am powerful, resilient and grateful.
I am powerful, resilient and grateful.
I am powerful, resilient and grateful.

Write your own:

I am _____

I am _____

I am _____

I am _____

I am _____

I am _____

I am _____

Remember to Visualise

DAY 17

**Find a peaceful place to read out loud the affirmations.
Repeat each paragraph 5 times, twice a day.**

I am attracting amazing opportunities into my life.
I am attracting amazing opportunities into my life.
I am attracting amazing opportunities into my life.

I am loved and appreciated. I am open to healthy and nurturing
relationships.
I am loved and appreciated. I am open to healthy and nurturing
relationships.
I am loved and appreciated. I am open to healthy and nurturing
relationships.

I am financially abundant and successful.
I am financially abundant and successful.
I am financially abundant and successful.

Write your own:

I am _____

I am _____

I am _____

I am _____

I am _____

I am _____

I am _____

DAY 18

Find a peaceful place to read out loud the affirmations.
Repeat each paragraph 5 times, twice a day.

II am in a great health and shape.
I am in a great health and shape.
I am in a great health and shape.

I am in love with my body, my person and my life.
I am in love with my body, my person and my life.
I am in love with my body, my person and my life.

I am always achieving my goals. I am a winner!
I am always achieving my goals. I am a winner!
I am always achieving my goals. I am a winner!

Write your own:

I am _____

I am _____

I am _____

I am _____

I am _____

I am _____

I am _____

DAY 19

Find a peaceful place to read out loud the affirmations.
Repeat each paragraph 5 times, twice a day.

I am manifesting powerful results in my life constantly.
I am manifesting powerful results in my life constantly.
I am manifesting powerful results in my life constantly.

I am attracting successful and great people to my life.
I am attracting successful and great people to my life.
I am attracting successful and great people to my life.

I am attracting a well-rewarded job opportunity.
I am attracting a well-rewarded job opportunity.
I am attracting a well-rewarded job opportunity.

Write your own:

I am _____

I am _____

I am _____

I am _____

I am _____

I am _____

I am _____

DAY 20

**Find a peaceful place to read out loud the affirmations.
Repeat each paragraph 5 times, twice a day.**

I am healthy, slim and strong.
I am healthy, slim and strong.
I am healthy, slim and strong.

I am amazing in what I do.
I am amazing in what I do.
I am amazing in what I do.

I am focused, persistent and will never quit.
I am focused, persistent and will never quit.
I am focused, persistent and will never quit.

Write your own:

I am _____

I am _____

I am _____

I am _____

I am _____

I am _____

I am _____

Remember to Visualise

REVIEW YOUR PROGRESS

Congratulations on being persistent on this 30-day challenge!

By this stage you should be able to see the changes in your life. Affirmations also helps to calm your body, release stress and give you large doses of confidence.

Remember to keep positive, combine the affirmations with visualisation as a powerful technique. The power is in your inner-self!

To add more power to the positive affirmation, write it down as you speak it.

Count your blessings and write down your achievements.

_____

_____

_____

_____

_____

DAY 21

Find a peaceful place to read out loud the affirmations.
Repeat each paragraph 5 times, twice a day.

I am always in control of my emotions and my thoughts.
I am always in control of my emotions and my thoughts.
I am always in control of my emotions and my thoughts.

I am capable of the impossible.
I am capable of the impossible.
I am capable of the impossible.

I am confident and courageous. I have the strength and the ability to accomplish my goals and dreams.
I am confident and courageous. I have the strength and the ability to accomplish my goals and dreams.
I am confident and courageous. I have the strength and the ability to accomplish my goals and dreams.

Write your own:

I am _____

I am _____

I am _____

I am _____

I am _____

I am _____

I am _____

DAY 22

Find a peaceful place to read out loud the affirmations.
Repeat each paragraph 5 times, twice a day.

II am fearless and powerful.
I am fearless and powerful.
I am fearless and powerful.

I am worthy of love and respect.
I am worthy of love and respect.
I am worthy of love and respect.

I am healthy and my body regenerates and rejuvenates every
second of my life.
I am healthy and my body regenerates and rejuvenates every
second of my life.
I am healthy and my body regenerates and rejuvenates every
second of my life.

Write your own:

I am _____

I am _____

I am _____

I am _____

I am _____

I am _____

I am _____

Remember to Visualise

DAY 23

Find a peaceful place to read out loud the affirmations.
Repeat each paragraph 5 times, twice a day.

II am positive, and I think positively.
I am positive, and I think positively.
I am positive, and I think positively.

I am in charge of how I feel, and I am feeling happy.
I am in charge of how I feel, and I am feeling happy.
I am in charge of how I feel, and I am feeling happy.

I am eating healthy, training hard and keeping myself inspired.
I am eating healthy, training hard and keeping myself inspired.
I am eating healthy, training hard and keeping myself inspired.

Write your own:

I am _____

I am _____

I am _____

I am _____

I am _____

I am _____

I am _____

DAY 24

**Find a peaceful place to read out loud the affirmations.
Repeat each paragraph 5 times, twice a day.**

I am blessed and grateful. I love my life.
I am blessed and grateful. I love my life.
I am blessed and grateful. I love my life.

I am an inspiration to others.
I am an inspiration to others.
I am an inspiration to others.

I am a money magnet and I am determined for greatness.
I am a money magnet and I am determined for greatness.
I am a money magnet and I am determined for greatness.

Write your own:

I am _____

I am _____

I am _____

I am _____

I am _____

I am _____

I am _____

DAY 25

Find a peaceful place to read out loud the affirmations.
Repeat each paragraph 5 times, twice a day.

I am talented, unique and admired.
I am talented, unique and admired.
I am talented, unique and admired.

I am brave, I am bold, I am strong.
I am brave, I am bold, I am strong.
I am brave, I am bold, I am strong.

I am always persisting in my objectives successfully.
I am always persisting in my objectives successfully.
I am always persisting in my objectives successfully.

Write your own:

I am _____

I am _____

I am _____

I am _____

I am _____

I am _____

I am _____

Remember to Visualise

DAY 26

**Find a peaceful place to read out loud the affirmations.
Repeat each paragraph 5 times, twice a day.**

I am always attracting the right moments and circumstances in my life.
I am always attracting the right moments and circumstances in my life.
I am always attracting the right moments and circumstances in my life.

I am incredible, assertive and resilient.
I am incredible, assertive and resilient.
I am incredible, assertive and resilient.

I am safe. I am divinely protected in all that I do.
I am safe. I am divinely protected in all that I do.
I am safe. I am divinely protected in all that I do.

Write your own:

I am _____

I am _____

I am _____

I am _____

I am _____

I am _____

I am _____

DAY 27

Find a peaceful place to read out loud the affirmations.
Repeat each paragraph 5 times, twice a day.

I am creative, innovative and smart.
I am creative, innovative and smart.
I am creative, innovative and smart.

I am considerate and create joy for others.
I am considerate and create joy for others.
I am considerate and create joy for others.

I am confident. I am powerful, and I will make it happen.
I am confident. I am powerful, and I will make it happen.
I am confident. I am powerful, and I will make it happen.

Write your own:

I am _____

I am _____

I am _____

I am _____

I am _____

I am _____

I am _____

DAY 28

**Find a peaceful place to read out loud the affirmations.
Repeat each paragraph 5 times, twice a day.**

I am who I am. I can do everything I set my mind to.
I am who I am. I can do everything I set my mind to.
I am who I am. I can do everything I set my mind to.

I am healed, I am forgiving, I am love.
I am healed, I am forgiving, I am love.
I am healed, I am forgiving, I am love.

I am worthy. I love every cell of my body.
I am worthy. I love every cell of my body.
I am worthy. I love every cell of my body.

Write your own:

I am _____

I am _____

I am _____

I am _____

I am _____

I am _____

I am _____

Remember to Visualise

DAY 29

**Find a peaceful place to read out loud the affirmations.
Repeat each paragraph 5 times, twice a day.**

I am grateful for every day of my life. I am capable of wonderful
things.
I am grateful for every day of my life. I am capable of wonderful
things.
I am grateful for every day of my life. I am capable of wonderful
things.

I am receiving successful outcomes, now and as I expected.
I am receiving successful outcomes, now and as I expected.
I am receiving successful outcomes, now and as I expected.

I am who I am. I am the way, the truth and my own life.
I am who I am. I am the way, the truth and my own life.
I am who I am. I am the way, the truth and my own life.

Write your own:

I am _____

I am _____

I am _____

I am _____

I am _____

I am _____

I am _____

DAY 30

**Find a peaceful place to read out loud the affirmations.
Repeat each paragraph 5 times, twice a day.**

I am different, unique and ready to receive the greatness of the universe.
I am different, unique and ready to receive the greatness of the universe.
I am different, unique and ready to receive the greatness of the universe.

I am who I am. I am here to be awesome.
I am who I am. I am here to be awesome.
I am who I am. I am here to be awesome.

I am part of the universe, fearless, possible and powerful.
I am part of the universe, fearless, possible and powerful.
I am part of the universe, fearless, possible and powerful.

Write your own:

I am _____

I am _____

I am _____

I am _____

I am _____

I am _____

I am _____

REVIEW YOUR PROGRESS

You are amazing! Congratulations on completing the 30 days powerful affirmation challenge!

Always keep in mind that a positive mental attitude supported by affirmations will achieve success in anything.

Feel free to repeat this journal any time, focusing on what you want to achieve. Keep it personal, keep it memorable!

Feel free to combine this technique with listening to positive affirmations audios.

Count your blessings and write down your achievements.

**Always follow your dreams.
You are in control of your life!**

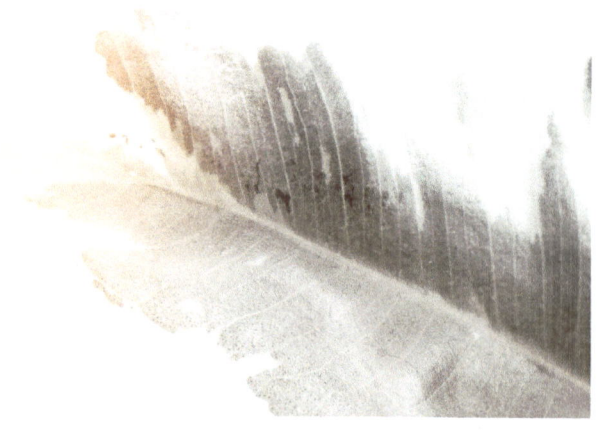

www.ingramcontent.com/pod-product-compliance
Lightning Source LLC
Chambersburg PA
CBHW050857290526
45792CB00002B/630